The Anti Inflammatory Diet Cookbook For Seniors

Easy and quick recipes to help improve your health as you age.

Mandy White

Copyright © 2023 By Mandy White.

Table of Contents

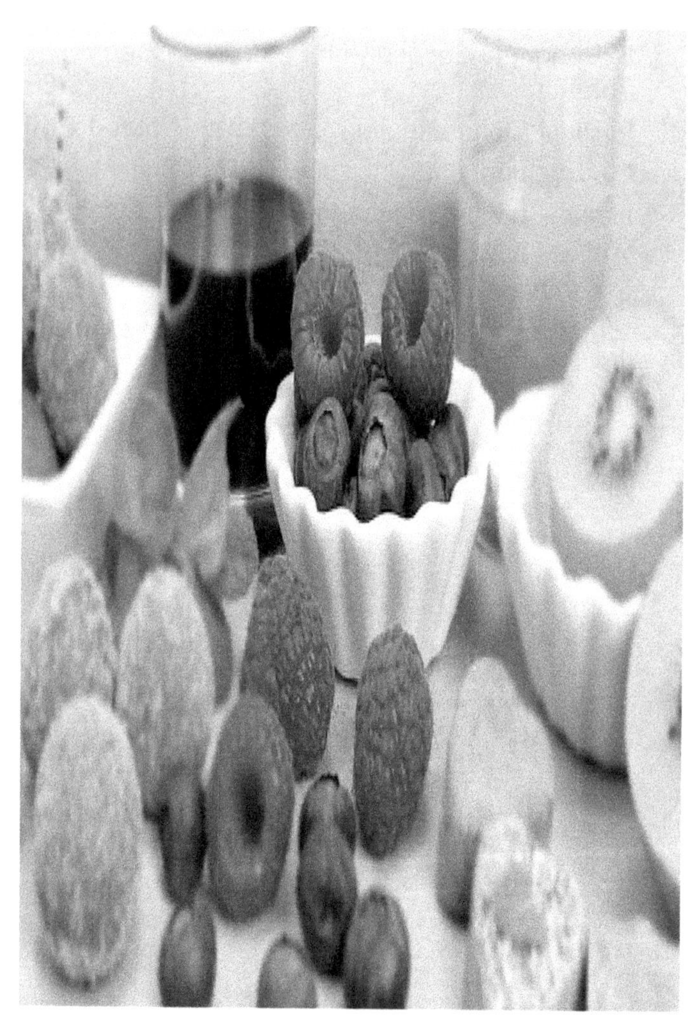

Introduction

My mother had spent a portion of her life battling a disorder that caused her ongoing pain and discomfort. Despite trying medications and treatments she hadn't found any long term relief.

One day she came across an article, in a health magazine that discussed the benefits of a diet in managing inflammatory disorders. This caught her interest so she decided to look into it. She consulted with a nutritionist who specializes in disorders and together they developed a meal plan for her.

My mother diligently followed the diet plan, which focused on foods, fruits, vegetables, lean proteins and healthy fats. She made sure to avoid processed foods, refined sugars and foods known to trigger inflammation. Initially it was challenging for her to adapt to this way of eating; however she remained determined.

Over the course of weeks she began noticing improvements in her condition. The constant pain started to decrease. Her energy levels started to rise. Encouraged by these changes she continued adhering to her dietary regimen.

Months passed, and her inflammatory disorder became more manageable than ever before. She no longer relied on heavy medications to alleviate her symptoms. Instead, she found solace in the healing power of nutritious food.

Words of her remarkable transformation spread throughout our neighborhood. People started seeking her advice, hoping to find relief from their own inflammatory disorders. She became a beacon of hope, sharing her knowledge and experiences with others.

With her new found purpose, my mum dedicated her time to educating her community about the importance of a healthy diet in managing inflammatory disorders. She organized workshops, cooking classes, and support groups, all aimed at empowering others to take control of their health. Seeing this great transformation in her, I decided to put together things that helped her manage her situation and share with others who find themselves in similar situations like she used to be; so they can also find help for themselves through reading this book and taking the right steps to a healthier life.

Chapter One

Understanding Inflammatory Disorders

Inflammatory disorders refer to a collection of conditions that involve inflammation, in areas of the body. Inflammation is a natural defense mechanism of the system designed to safeguard the body against substances like pathogens, injuries or irritants. However sometimes the immune system can become excessively reactive and initiate inflammation, even in the absence of an obvious danger. This can result in ceaseless inflammation and the emergence of inflammatory disorders.

Various Forms of Inflammatory Disorders

Numerous types of disorders exist,each affecting different parts of the body. Some common examples include:

1. Rheumatoid arthritis: This is an autoimmune disorder that primarily affects the joints, causing pain, stiffness, and swelling. This takes place as a result of the immune system mistakenly attacking the body's tissues, causing chronic inflammation of the joints.

2. Inflammatory bowel disease (IBD): This includes conditions like Crohn's disease and ulcerative colitis, which cause inflammation in the digestive tract. This often appears with symptoms like, diarrhea, abdominal discomfort, fatigue and weight loss.

3. Asthma: Asthma is a chronic inflammatory disorder of the airways, leading to symptoms such as wheezing, coughing, shortness of breath, and chest tightness.

4. Psoriasis: Psoriasis is a skin disorder characterized by red, scaly patches on the skin. It occurs due to an overactive immune response, leading to inflammation and rapid skin cell turnover.

5. Chronic obstructive pulmonary disease (COPD): COPD is a progressive lung disease that causes inflammation in the airways, leading to breathing difficulties. This is usually a resultant effect of long term exposure to irritants like tobacco smoke

Causes of Inflammatory Disorder:

The causes of inflammatory disorders can vary depending on the specific condition. In some cases, genetic factors may play a role, making certain individuals more susceptible to developing these disorders. Environmental factors, such as exposure to pollutants or certain infections, can also contribute to the development of inflammation.

Symptoms of Inflammatory Disorders

The symptoms of inflammatory disorders can vary widely depending on the affected area of the body. However, some common symptoms include pain, swelling, redness, heat, and loss of function in the affected area. Systemic symptoms such as fatigue, fever, and weight loss may also occur in some cases.

Managing Inflammatory Disorders

Inflammatory disorders can be managed and prevented through various measures. Here are some preventive measures that can help reduce the risk of inflammatory disorders:

1. Maintain a healthy diet: Consuming a balanced diet rich in fruits, vegetables, whole grains, and lean proteins can help reduce inflammation in the body. Avoiding processed foods, sugary drinks, and excessive alcohol consumption is also beneficial.

2. Regular exercise: Engaging in regular physical activity can help reduce inflammation and improve overall health. Engage in at least 75-150 minutes of energetic exercise weekly

3. Manage stress: Chronic stress can contribute to inflammation. Engage in stress management techniques like, deep breathing exercises, meditation or other activities you delight in to help minimize stress levels.

4. Get enough sleep: As we discussed earlier, getting enough sleep is important for overall health. Lack of sleep can increase inflammation in the body, so aim for 7-9 hours of quality sleep each night.

5. Maintain a healthy weight: Being overweight or obese can increase inflammation in the body. Adopting a healthy lifestyle that includes regular exercise and a balanced diet can help maintain a healthy weight and reduce inflammation.

6. Avoid smoking: Smoking is a major contributor to inflammation and various health problems. Quitting smoking or avoiding exposure to secondhand smoke can significantly reduce the risk of inflammatory disorders.

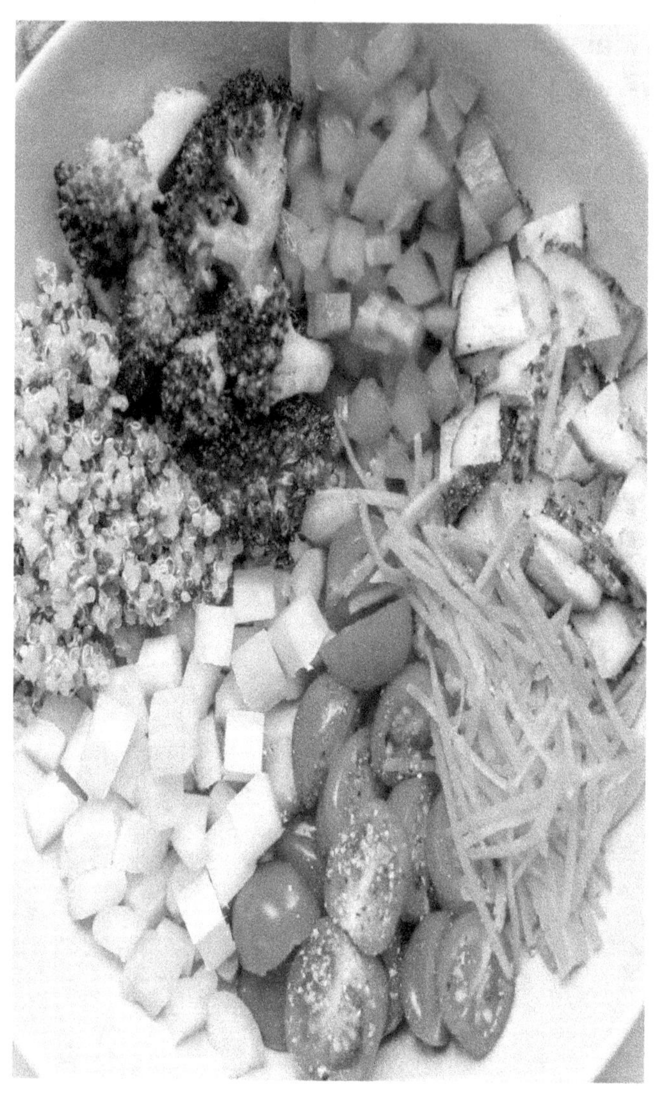

Chapter Two

Diets for Anti Inflammatory Disorders.

What to Eat and What not to Eat

An inflammatory disorder diet aims to reduce inflammation in the body and promote overall health.

Foods to eat on an inflammatory disorder diet:

1. Fruits and vegetables: These are rich in antioxidants, vitamins, and minerals that can help reduce inflammation. Go for a combination of colorful fruits and vegetables.

2. Whole grains: Opt for whole grains like brown rice, quinoa, and whole wheat bread, as they contain more fiber and nutrients compared to refined grains.

3. Healthy fats: Include sources of healthy fats such as avocados, olive oil, nuts, and seeds. They contain anti-inflammatory properties which can boost overall health.

4. Fatty fish: Fish like salmon, mackerel, and sardines are high in omega-3 fatty acids, which have been shown to reduce inflammation.

5. Legumes: Beans, lentils, and chickpeas are excellent sources of plant-based protein and fiber, and they can help reduce inflammation.

6. Herbs and spices: Turmeric, ginger, garlic, cloves and cinnamon have anti-inflammatory properties and can be beneficial when added to meals.

Foods to Avoid on an Inflammatory Disorder Diet:

1. Processed foods: These often contain high levels of unhealthy fats, added sugars, and artificial additives, which can promote inflammation. Examples include fast food, packaged snacks, and sugary drinks.

2. Trans fats: Found in fried foods, margarine, and many processed baked goods, trans fats can increase inflammation and should be avoided.

3. Refined carbohydrates: Foods like white bread, white rice, and sugary cereals can cause spikes in blood sugar levels and promote inflammation.

4. Red and processed meats: High consumption of red and processed meats has been linked to increased inflammation. Cut down their consumption and go for leaner protein sources.

5. High-sugar foods: Excessive sugar intake can lead to chronic inflammation. Stay away from sweetened beverages and desserts, sodas, and their likes.

6. Alcohol: While moderate alcohol consumption may not be harmful, excessive intake can contribute to inflammation and other health issues.

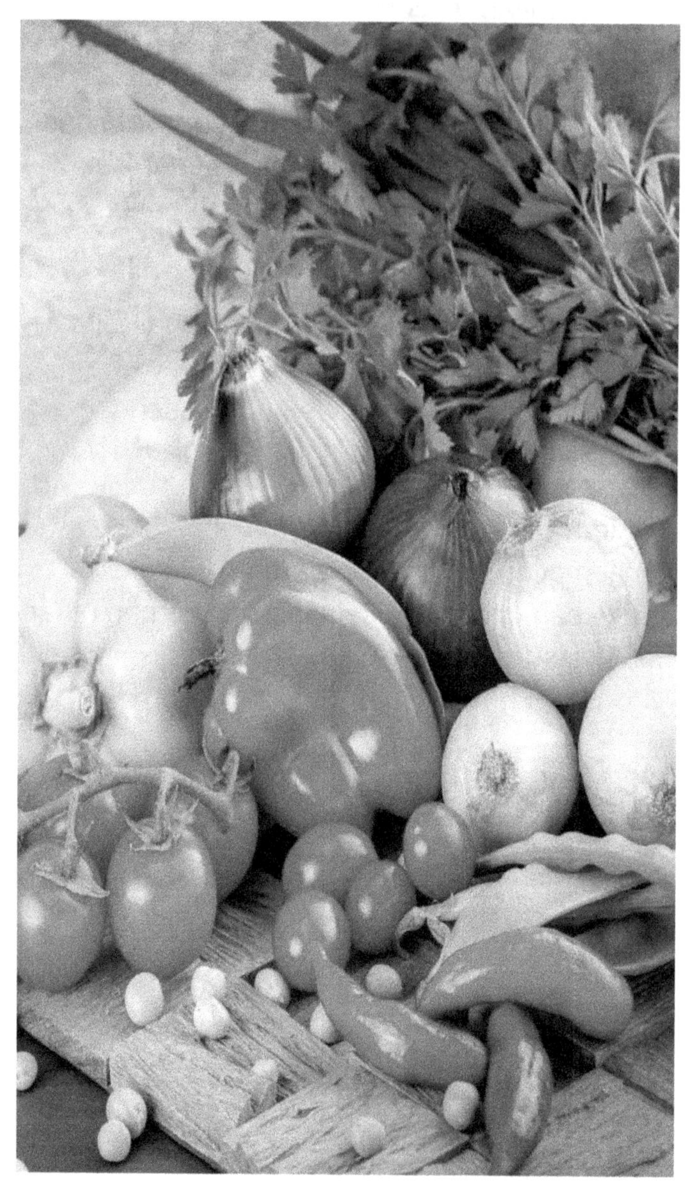

Chapter Three

Advantages of Anti Inflammatory Diet

Following an inflammatory disorder diet can have several core benefits for seniors. Here are some of them:

1. Reduced inflammation: An inflammatory disorder diet focuses on consuming foods that have anti-inflammatory properties. By following this diet, you can help reduce inflammation in your body, which can be beneficial for managing conditions like arthritis, asthma, or inflammatory bowel disease.

2. Improved digestion: Inflammatory disorder diets must include whole, unprocessed foods that are rich in fiber. This can help improve digestion and promote a healthy gut, which is important for overall well-being.

3. Weight management: Inflammatory disorder diets often encourage the consumption of nutrient-dense foods while limiting processed foods and added sugars. This can help with weight management and maintaining a healthy body weight.

4. Enhanced immune function: Certain foods included in an inflammatory disorder diet, such as fruits, vegetables, and lean proteins, are known to support a healthy immune system. By following this diet, you can potentially boost your immune function and reduce the risk of infections.

5. Increased energy levels: A diet that focuses on whole, nutrient-rich foods can provide your body with the necessary fuel to function optimally. This can improve energy levels and boost overall vitality.

Note: It's important to note that the specific benefits may vary depending on individual circumstances and the specific inflammatory disorder.

Chapter Four

Complications that come with inflammatory disorders:

Inflammatory disorders can lead to a range of complications if the right diet and appropriate medical management are not adopted. While the specifics can vary depending on the type and severity of the inflammatory condition, here are some common complications associated with untreated or poorly managed inflammatory disorders:

1. Chronic Inflammation: Failure to address inflammation with dietary and lifestyle changes can lead to chronic inflammation, which is associated with a host of health issues. Chronic inflammation is thought to contribute to various conditions, including heart disease, diabetes, and cancer.

2. Progression of the Underlying Condition: Many inflammatory disorders are chronic, progressive diseases. Without proper management, the underlying condition may worsen over time, causing increased pain, discomfort, and complications.

3. Tissue Damage: Inflammatory disorders often result in tissue damage. Continued inflammation can lead to the destruction of affected tissues or organs, causing permanent damage and impairing their function.

4. Joint Damage: Inflammatory joint disorders like rheumatoid arthritis, if not managed well, can lead to joint damage and deformities, affecting mobility and quality of life.

5. Cardiovascular Issues: Chronic inflammation can damage blood vessels and increase the risk of cardiovascular diseases like atherosclerosis (hardening of the arteries) and hypertension (high blood pressure).

6. Gastrointestinal Problems: Inflammatory bowel diseases (IBD), including Crohn's disease and ulcerative colitis, can lead to severe complications like intestinal obstructions, malnutrition, and even an increased risk of colon cancer when not properly managed.

7. Kidney Problems: Inflammatory disorders can affect kidney function, potentially leading to kidney disease or even kidney failure if left uncontrolled.

8. Autoimmune Complications: Inflammatory disorders often involve autoimmune responses. If these responses are not regulated, they can result in damage to healthy tissues and organs.

9. Mental Health Impacts: Living with chronic inflammation and the complications it brings can take a toll on mental health. Conditions like depression and anxiety are more common in individuals with chronic inflammatory disorders.

10. Reduced Quality of Life: Uncontrolled inflammation can result in a lower quality of life due to persistent pain, fatigue, mobility issues, and other symptoms that impact daily activities and overall wellbeing.

Chapter Five

Meal Planning Benefits

Meal planning for an inflammatory disorders diet involves selecting foods that have anti-inflammatory properties and avoiding foods that can trigger inflammation. The benefits of proper meal planning for managing inflammatory disorders include:

1. Reduced inflammation: A well-planned diet can help reduce inflammation in the body by including foods that have anti-inflammatory properties, such as fruits, vegetables, whole grains, fatty fish, nuts, and seeds.

2. Balanced nutrient intake: Meal planning ensures that you are getting a balanced intake of essential nutrients, including vitamins, minerals, and antioxidants, which are important for managing inflammation and supporting overall health.

3. Weight management: A carefully planned diet can help with weight management, which is crucial for managing inflammatory disorders. Maintaining a healthy weight can help reduce inflammation and improve symptoms.

4. Improved gut health: Meal planning can include foods that promote a healthy gut microbiome, which plays a role in managing inflammation. Foods like probiotics (found in yogurt and fermented foods) and prebiotics (found in fruits, vegetables, and whole grains) can support gut health.

24 Day-Meal Plan

Below is a meal plan guide to help you manage and improve your health.

DAY 1:

Breakfast: Greek yogurt with honey and berries.

Lunch: Quinoa salad with spinach, cherry tomatoes, cucumber, and a lemon-tahini dressing.

Dinner: Baked salmon with asparagus and a side of quinoa.

Day 2:

Breakfast: Scrambled eggs with sautéed spinach and sliced avocado.

Lunch: Lentil soup with a side of mixed greens.

Dinner: Grilled chicken breast with roasted sweet potatoes and steamed broccoli.

Day 3:

Breakfast: Oatmeal with chia seeds, almond butter, and sliced bananas.

Lunch: Tuna salad with mixed greens, olives, and a balsamic vinaigrette.

Dinner: Baked cod with a side of quinoa and grilled zucchini.

Day 4:

Breakfast: Smoothie with kale, pineapple, ginger, and flaxseeds.

Lunch: Brown rice bowl with black beans, roasted red peppers, and avocado.

Dinner: Turkey meatballs with whole wheat pasta and a tomato-basil sauce.

Day 5

Breakfast: Whole grain toast with almond butter and sliced strawberries.

Lunch: Mixed bean salad with bell peppers, red onion, and a lemon-olive oil dressing.

Dinner: Grilled shrimp with quinoa and sautéed kale.

Day 6:

Breakfast: Cottage cheese with sliced peaches and a drizzle of honey.

Lunch: Spinach and arugula salad with grilled chicken, cherry tomatoes, and a homemade vinaigrette.

Dinner: Baked tofu with brown rice and stir-fried bok choy.

Day 7:

Breakfast: Whole grain waffles with fresh berries and Greek yogurt.

Lunch: Miso soup with seaweed and tofu, and a side of steamed edamame.

Dinner: Roasted vegetable and quinoa-stuffed bell peppers.

Breakfast: Overnight oats made with almond milk, chia seeds, and mixed berries.

Lunch: Spinach and kale salad with grilled tempeh, roasted beets, and a tahini dressing.

Dinner: Baked white fish with a side of quinoa and steamed asparagus.

Breakfast: A smoothie with spinach, pineapple, mango, and a touch of ginger.

Lunch: Lentil and vegetable stew with a side of mixed greens.

Dinner: Grilled chicken breast with a warm quinoa and roasted vegetable salad.

Breakfast: Scrambled eggs with sautéed mushrooms and sliced avocado.

Lunch: Chickpea and kale salad with lemon-tahini dressing.

Dinner: Baked salmon with a side of wild rice and grilled zucchini.

Day 11:

Breakfast: Greek yogurt with honey, sliced banana, and a sprinkle of ground flaxseeds.

Lunch: Mixed greens with grilled shrimp, cherry tomatoes, and a balsamic vinaigrette.

Dinner: Baked tofu with quinoa and steamed broccoli.

Day 12:

Breakfast: Oatmeal with almond butter, sliced strawberries, and a drizzle of honey.

Lunch: Brown rice bowl with black beans, corn, and avocado.

Dinner: Grilled turkey burger with sweet potato wedges and sautéed spinach.

Day 13:

Breakfast: Smoothie with kale, blueberries, banana, and a spoon of flaxseed.

Lunch: Spinach and arugula salad with grilled chicken, mixed berries, and a raspberry vinaigrette.

Dinner: Baked cod with a side of quinoa and roasted Brussels sprouts.

Day 14:

Breakfast: Whole grain toast with avocado slices and a poached egg.

Lunch: Lentil soup with a side of mixed greens and sliced cucumber.

Dinner: Grilled vegetable and quinoa-stuffed bell peppers.

Day 15:

Breakfast: Oatmeal topped with berries and a sprinkle of walnuts

Lunch: Grilled chicken salad with mixed greens, cherry tomatoes, cucumber, and olive oil dressing

Snack: Carrot sticks with hummus

Dinner: Baked salmon with roasted vegetables (broccoli, bell peppers, and sweet potatoes)

Dessert: Greek yogurt with honey and sliced almonds

Breakfast: Spinach and mushroom omelette with whole grain toast

Lunch: Quinoa salad with mixed vegetables, chickpeas, and lemon vinaigrette

Snack: Apple slices with almond butter

Dinner: Grilled tofu with stir-fried vegetables (bell peppers, snap peas, and carrots) and brown rice

Dessert: Mixed berries with a dollop of coconut cream

Day 17:

Breakfast: Avocado toast on whole grain bread with a side of sliced tomatoes

Lunch: Lentil soup with a side of mixed green salad

Snack: Greek yogurt with chia seeds and a drizzle of honey

Dinner: Grilled chicken breast with steamed broccoli and quinoa

Dessert: Dark chocolate squares

Breakfast: chia pudding with berries and nuts.

Lunch: grilled chicken, cherry tomatoes, avocado and spinach salad with lemon-turmeric dressing.

Grilled salmon with roasted Brussels sprouts and quinoa.

Day 19:

Breakfast: Oatmeal with almond milk, sliced bananas and a drizzle of honey.

Lunch: Quinoa and black bean salad with crushed peppers, cucumber and lime cilantro dressing.

Dinner: grilled chicken breast, steamed broccoli and brown rice.

Day 20:

Breakfast: Greek yogurt with mixed berries, a spoonful of almond butter and a pinch of flax seeds.

Lunch: Green salad mixed with lentil soup and topped with roasted chickpeas.

Dinner: Baked tofu with quinoa and steamed broccoli.

Breakfast: Smoked salmon and avocado on whole grain toast.

Lunch: Mediterranean salad with mixed greens, olives, feta cheese, cherry tomatoes, and a lemon-olive oil dressing.

Dinner: Grilled shrimp skewers with grilled vegetables and quinoa.

Breakfast: Green smoothie made with spinach, pineapple, banana, and coconut milk.

Lunch: Baked sweet potato topped with black beans, salsa, and a dollop of Greek yogurt.

Dinner: Grilled chicken skewers with a side of roasted cauliflower and brown rice.

Breakfast: Quinoa porridge cooked with almond milk, topped with sliced peaches and a sprinkle of cinnamon.

Lunch: Spinach and quinoa salad with roasted beets, goat cheese, and a balsamic dressing.

Dinner: Baked tofu with stir-fried vegetables and brown rice.

Day 24:

Breakfast: Omelette made with egg whites, spinach, mushrooms, and a sprinkle of feta cheese.

Lunch: Quinoa and roasted vegetable salad with bell peppers, zucchini, cherry tomatoes, and a lemon-tahini dressing.

Dinner: Grilled salmon with steamed asparagus and wild rice.

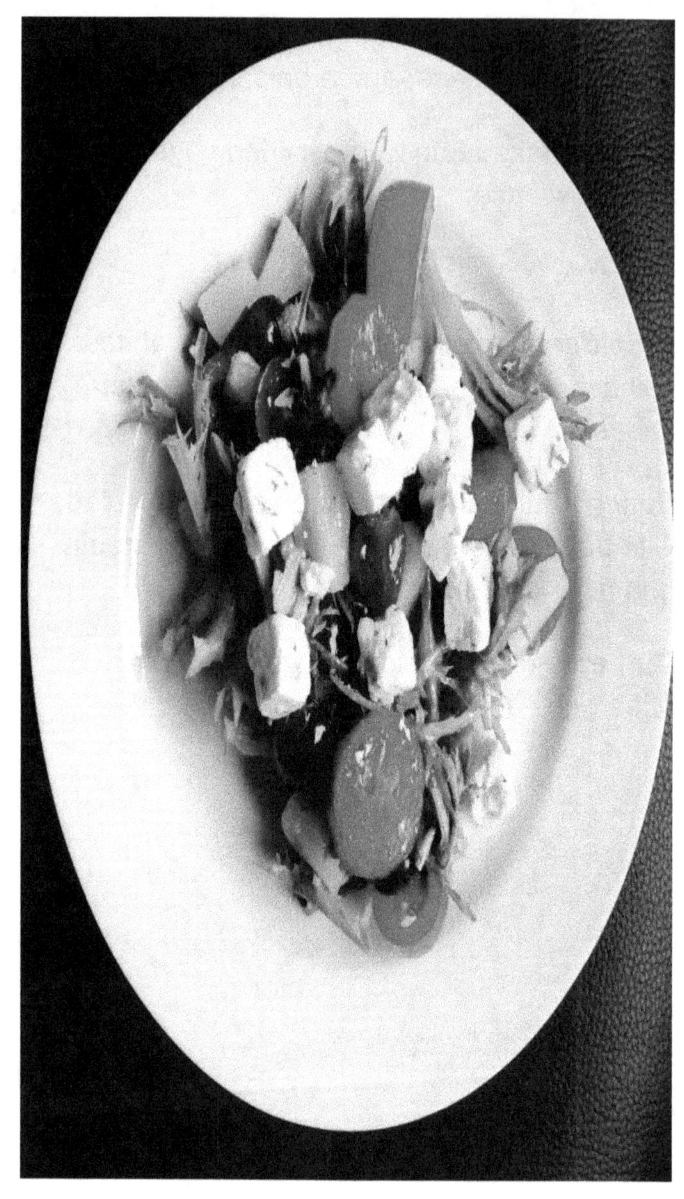

Chapter Six

Anti inflammatory diet recipes for breakfast, lunch and dinner, preparation methods, cooking time and their nutritional values

10 Breakfast Recipes

Here are 10 anti-inflammatory disorder diet breakfast recipes along with their ingredients, preparation methods, quantity or measurements, nutritional value, and estimated cooking times:

1. Berry and Spinach Smoothie Bowl

Ingredients:

1 cup fresh spinach

1/2 cup mixed berries (strawberries, blueberries, raspberries)

1/2 banana

1/2 cup Greek yogurt

1 tablespoon chia seeds

Preparation:

1. Blend spinach, mixed berries, banana, and Greek yogurt until smooth.

2. Pour the mixture into a bowl and top with chia seeds.

Nutritional Value: High in fiber, antioxidants, and vitamins.

Cooking Time: 5 minutes.

2. Avocado and Salmon Toast

Ingredients:

1/2 avocado, mashed

2 slices whole-grain bread

4 oz smoked salmon

Fresh dill for garnish

Preparation:

1. Toast the whole-grain bread slices.

2. Spread mashed avocado on the toast and top with smoked salmon.

3. Garnish with fresh dill.

Nutritional Value: Rich in omega-3 fatty acids and healthy fats.

Cooking Time: 5 minutes.

3. Turmeric Scrambled Eggs

Ingredients:

2 eggs

1/4 teaspoon turmeric powder

1/4 teaspoon black pepper

Chopped fresh parsley for garnish

Preparation:

1. Whisk eggs with turmeric and black pepper.

2. Cook the eggs in a non-stick pan until scrambled.

3. Garnish with chopped fresh parsley.

Nutritional Value: Anti-inflammatory turmeric and protein.

Cooking Time: 5 minutes.

4. Greek Yogurt Parfait

Ingredients:

1 cup Greek yogurt

1/2 cup fresh berries (e.g., blueberries, raspberries)

1/4 cup granola (low sugar)

Honey (optional)

Preparation:

1. Layer Greek yogurt, fresh berries, and granola in a glass.

2. Drizzle with honey if desired.

Nutritional Value: Protein, probiotics, and antioxidants.

Cooking Time: 2 minutes.

5. Chia Seed Pudding

Ingredients:

2 tablespoons chia seeds

1 cup unsweetened almond milk

1/2 teaspoon pure vanilla extract

Fresh fruit for topping (e.g., sliced banana, kiwi)

Preparation:

1. Mix chia seeds, almond milk, and vanilla extract in a jar or bowl.

2. Refrigerate overnight or for at least 3 hours until it thickens.

3. Top with fresh fruit before serving.

Nutritional Value: Omega-3 fatty acids, fiber, and vitamins.

Cooking Time: No cooking, but requires soaking.

6. Quinoa Breakfast Bowl

Ingredients:

1/2 cup cooked quinoa

1/4 cup almond milk

Sliced peaches or other fresh fruit

Chopped nuts (e.g., almonds, walnuts)

Honey (optional)

Preparation:

1. Heat cooked quinoa with almond milk until warm.

2. Top with fresh fruit, chopped nuts, and a drizzle of honey.

Nutritional Value: Protein, fiber, and vitamins.

Cooking Time: 5 minutes.

7. Sweet Potato and Spinach Omelette.

Ingredients:

2 eggs

1/2 cup cooked sweet potato, diced

1 cup fresh spinach

1/4 cup diced bell peppers

A pinch of turmeric

Preparation:

1. Whisk eggs with a pinch of turmeric.

2. In a non-stick pan, sauté sweet potato, bell peppers, and spinach until tender.

3. Pour the eggs over the vegetables and cook until set.

Nutritional Value: Protein, fiber, antioxidants, and vitamins.

Cooking Time: 10 minutes.

8. Peanut Butter Banana Toast.

Ingredients:

2 slices whole-grain bread

2 tablespoons natural peanut butter

1 banana, sliced

Preparation:

1. Toast the whole-grain bread slices.

2. Spread peanut butter on the toast and top with banana slices.

Nutritional Value: Healthy fats, protein, and potassium.

Cooking Time: 5 minutes.

9. Spinach and Feta Breakfast Wrap.

Ingredients:

2 eggs, scrambled

1 cup fresh spinach

2 tablespoons crumbled feta cheese

1 whole-grain tortilla

Preparation:

1. Scramble the eggs in a non-stick pan.

2. Place scrambled eggs, fresh spinach, and feta cheese on a tortilla.

3. Roll it into a wrap.

Nutritional Value: Protein, fiber, and calcium.

Cooking Time: 5 minutes.

10. Oatmeal with Almonds and Berries.

Ingredients:

1/2 cup rolled oats

1 cup almond milk

2 tablespoons slivered almonds

1/4 cup mixed berries

A drizzle of honey (optional)

Preparation:

1. Cook rolled oats with almond milk until creamy.

2. Top with slivered almonds, mixed berries, and honey if desired.

Nutritional Value: Fiber, antioxidants, and healthy fats.

Cooking Time: 10 minutes.

10 Lunch Recipes

10 anti-inflammatory disorder diet lunch recipes along with their ingredients, preparation methods, quantity or measurements, nutritional value, and estimated cooking times:

1. Quinoa and Chickpea Salad

Ingredients:

1 cup cooked quinoa

1 cup canned chickpeas, drained and rinsed

1 cup diced cucumber

1/2 cup cherry tomatoes, halved

1/4 cup chopped fresh parsley

2 tablespoons olive oil

2 tablespoons lemon juice

Salt and pepper to taste

Preparation:

1. In a bowl, combine quinoa, chickpeas, cucumber, cherry tomatoes, and fresh parsley.

2. In a separate bowl, whisk together olive oil and lemon juice, then drizzle over the salad.

3. Toss the salad gently to combine, and season with salt and pepper.

4. Serve chilled.

Nutritional Value: High in fiber, protein, antioxidants, and healthy fats.

Cooking Time: 15 minutes.

2. Grilled Chicken and Vegetable Wrap

Ingredients:

4 oz grilled chicken breast, sliced

1 whole-grain tortilla

1/4 cup sliced bell peppers

1/4 cup sliced zucchini

1/4 cup baby spinach

2 tablespoons hummus

Preparation:

1. Lay the tortilla flat and spread hummus evenly.

2. Layer grilled chicken, bell peppers, zucchini, and baby spinach.

3. Roll it into a wrap.

Nutritional Value: Lean protein, fiber, vitamins, and antioxidants.

Cooking Time: 15 minutes (for grilling the chicken).

3. Lentil and Vegetable Stir-Fry

Ingredients:

1 cup cooked brown lentils

1 cup broccoli florets

1/2 cup bell peppers, sliced

1/2 cup sliced carrots

1/4 cup low-sodium soy sauce

1 tablespoon sesame oil

1 teaspoon ginger, minced

Preparation:

1. In a wok or large pan, heat sesame oil and sauté ginger.

2. Add broccoli, bell peppers, and carrots, and stir-fry until tender.

3. Add cooked lentils and soy sauce, and cook for a few more minutes.

4. Serve hot.

Nutritional Value: High in fiber, plant-based protein, and antioxidants.

Cooking Time: 20 minutes.

4. Salmon and Quinoa Bowl

Ingredients:

4 oz baked or grilled salmon

1 cup cooked quinoa

1 cup steamed asparagus

1/4 cup diced avocado

1 tablespoon olive oil

1 tablespoon lemon juice

Fresh dill for garnish

Preparation:

1. Place quinoa in a bowl and top with salmon, steamed asparagus, and diced avocado.

2. Drizzle with olive oil and lemon juice.

3. Garnish with fresh dill.

Nutritional Value: Omega-3 fatty acids, protein, fiber, vitamins, and healthy fats.

Cooking Time: 20 minutes (for baking or grilling salmon).

5. Mediterranean Chickpea Salad

Ingredients:

1 can (15 oz) chickpeas, drained and rinsed

1 cucumber, diced

1 cup cherry tomatoes, halved

1/2 cup diced red onion

1/4 cup chopped fresh parsley

2 tablespoons extra-virgin olive oil

2 tablespoons red wine vinegar

1 teaspoon dried oregano

Salt and pepper to taste

Preparation:

1. In a large bowl, combine chickpeas, cucumber, cherry tomatoes, red onion, and fresh parsley.

2. In a separate bowl, whisk together olive oil, red wine vinegar, dried oregano, salt, and pepper.

3. Drizzle the dressing over the salad and toss to combine.

4. Serve chilled.

Nutritional Value: High in fiber, plant-based protein, antioxidants, and healthy fats.

Cooking Time: No cooking required.

6. Turkey and Vegetable Stir-Fry

Ingredients:

4 oz ground turkey

1 cup mixed stir-fry vegetables (e.g., bell peppers, broccoli, snap peas)

1 tablespoon low-sodium soy sauce

1 teaspoon ginger, minced

1 teaspoon garlic, minced

Preparation:

1. In a pan, cook ground turkey until browned.

2. Remove turkey from the pan and set aside.

3. In the same pan, stir-fry mixed vegetables, ginger, and garlic until tender.

4. Add the cooked turkey and soy sauce, and cook for a few more minutes.

5. Serve hot.

Nutritional Value: Lean protein, fiber, antioxidants, and low in saturated fats.

Cooking Time: 15 minutes.

7. Spinach and Quinoa Stuffed Bell Peppers

Ingredients:

2 bell peppers

1 cup cooked quinoa

1 cup fresh spinach, chopped

1/2 cup canned black beans, drained and rinsed

1/4 cup diced tomatoes

1/4 cup shredded mozzarella cheese (optional)

1/2 teaspoon cumin

Salt and pepper to taste

Preparation:

1. Preheat the oven to 375°F (190°C).

2. Cut the tops off the bell peppers and remove seeds.

3. In a bowl, combine cooked quinoa, chopped spinach, black beans, diced tomatoes, cumin, salt, and pepper.

4. Stuff the bell peppers with the quinoa mixture.

5. If desired, sprinkle mozzarella cheese on top.

6. Bake for 25-30 minutes until peppers are tender.

Nutritional Value: Fiber, protein, vitamins, and antioxidants.

Cooking Time:35 minutes.

8. Tomato and Basil Quinoa Salad

Ingredients:

1 cup cooked quinoa

1 cup cherry tomatoes, halved

1/2 cup fresh basil leaves, chopped

1/4 cup crumbled feta cheese

2 tablespoons balsamic vinaigrette

Salt and pepper to taste

Preparation:

1. In a bowl, combine cooked quinoa, cherry tomatoes, fresh basil, and crumbled feta cheese.

2. Drizzle with balsamic vinaigrette, and season with salt and pepper.

3. Toss to combine and serve.

Nutritional Value: Protein, fiber, antioxidants,

9. Black Bean and Sweet Potato Quesadilla

Ingredients:

1 whole-grain tortilla

1/2 cup canned black beans, drained and rinsed

1/2 cup cooked sweet potato, mashed

1/4 cup shredded cheddar cheese

1/4 cup diced red onion

1/2 teaspoon cumin

1/2 teaspoon chili powder

Olive oil for cooking

Preparation:

1. In a bowl, mix black beans, mashed sweet potato, shredded cheddar cheese, diced red onion, cumin, and chili powder.

2. Spread the mixture onto half of the tortilla, then fold the other half over it.

3. In a pan, heat a small amount of olive oil.

4. Cook the quesadilla until both sides are golden and the cheese is melted.

5. Slice and serve.

Nutritional Value: Protein, fiber, vitamins, and antioxidants.

Cooking Time: 10 minutes.

10. Tuna and Avocado Salad

Ingredients:

1 can (5 oz) canned tuna, drained

1 ripe avocado, diced

1/4 cup red bell pepper, diced

1/4 cup red onion, diced

1 tablespoon olive oil

1 tablespoon lemon juice

Fresh parsley for garnish

Preparation:

1. In a bowl, combine canned tuna, diced avocado, red bell pepper, and red onion.

2. Drizzle with olive oil and lemon juice.

3. Garnish with fresh parsley.

Nutritional Value: Lean protein, healthy fats, fiber, and vitamins.

No cooking required.

10 Dinner recipes

1. Baked Salmon with Quinoa and Asparagus

Ingredients:

4 oz salmon fillet

1/2 cup quinoa

1 cup asparagus spears

1 lemon

1 tablespoon olive oil

Fresh dill for garnish

Salt and pepper to taste

Preparation:

1. Preheat the oven to 375°F (190°C).

2. Season the salmon with olive oil, lemon juice, salt, and pepper.

3. Place the salmon on a baking sheet and add asparagus spears.

4. Bake for 15-20 minutes until salmon is cooked.

5. While baking, cook quinoa according to package instructions.

6. Serve salmon over cooked quinoa, garnished with fresh dill.

Nutritional Value: Omega-3 fatty acids, protein, fiber, and vitamins.

Cooking Time: 20-25 minutes.

2. Grilled Chicken with Roasted Vegetables

Ingredients:

4 oz grilled chicken breast

1 cup mixed roasted vegetables (e.g., bell peppers, zucchini, cherry tomatoes)

1 tablespoon olive oil

Fresh rosemary for garnish

Salt and pepper to taste

Preparation:

1. Grill the chicken breast until fully cooked.

2. Toss mixed vegetables with olive oil, salt, and pepper.

3. Roast the vegetables in the oven at 375°F (190°C) for 20 minutes.

4. Serve the grilled chicken over the roasted vegetables, garnished with fresh rosemary.

Nutritional Value: Lean protein, fiber, antioxidants, and vitamins.

Cooking Time: 30 minutes (including grilling and roasting).

3. Quinoa and Black Bean Stuffed Bell Peppers.

Ingredients:

2 bell peppers

1 cup cooked quinoa

1 cup canned black beans, drained and rinsed

1/2 cup diced tomatoes

1/4 cup shredded cheddar cheese

1/2 teaspoon cumin

1/2 teaspoon chili powder

Preparation:

1. Preheat the oven to 375°F (190°C).

2. Cut the tops off the bell peppers and remove seeds.

3. In a bowl, mix quinoa, black beans, diced tomatoes, cheddar cheese, cumin, and chili powder.

4. Stuff the bell peppers with the quinoa mixture.

5. Bake for 25-30 minutes until peppers are tender.

Nutritional Value: Protein, fiber, vitamins, and antioxidants.

Cooking Time: 35 minutes.

4. Sautéed Shrimp with Broccoli and Brown Rice.

Ingredients:

4 oz shrimp, peeled and deveined

1 cup broccoli florets

1/2 cup cooked brown rice

1 tablespoon olive oil

1 clove garlic, minced

1/2 lemon

Salt and pepper to taste

Preparation:

1. In a pan, heat olive oil and sauté garlic until fragrant.

2. Add shrimp and cook until they turn pink.

3. Remove shrimp from the pan and set aside.

4. Sauté broccoli until tender.

5. Serve shrimp and broccoli over cooked brown rice.

6. Squeeze lemon juice over the dish, and season with salt and pepper.

Nutritional Value: Protein, fiber, vitamins, and antioxidants.

Cooking Time: 15 minutes.

5. Vegetable and Tofu Stir-Fry

Ingredients:

4 oz firm tofu, cubed

1 cup mixed stir-fry vegetables (e.g., bell peppers, broccoli, snap peas)

2 tablespoons low-sodium soy sauce

1 tablespoon sesame oil

1 teaspoon ginger, minced

1 teaspoon garlic, minced

Preparation:

1. In a pan, heat sesame oil and sauté ginger and garlic.

2. Add tofu cubes and cook until lightly browned.

3. Remove tofu from the pan and set aside.

4. Stir-fry mixed vegetables until tender.

5. Add tofu and soy sauce to the pan, and cook for a few more minutes.

6. Serve hot.

Nutritional Value: Plant-based protein, fiber, antioxidants, and vitamins.

Cooking Time: 20 minutes.

6. Mediterranean Chickpea Salad with Grilled Chicken

Ingredients:

4 oz grilled chicken breast, sliced

1 can (15 oz) canned chickpeas, drained and rinsed

1 cucumber, diced

1 cup cherry tomatoes, halved

1/4 cup chopped fresh parsley

2 tablespoons extra-virgin olive oil

2 tablespoons red wine vinegar

1 teaspoon dried oregano

Salt and pepper to taste

Preparation:

1. In a bowl, combine chickpeas, cucumber, cherry tomatoes, fresh parsley.

2. In a separate bowl, whisk together olive oil, red wine vinegar, dried oregano, salt, and pepper.

3. Drizzle the dressing over the salad.

4. Top the salad with grilled chicken slices.

5. Serve chilled.

Nutritional Value: Lean protein, fiber, antioxidants, and healthy fats.

Cooking Time: 20 minutes (including grilling).

7. Sweet Potato and Lentil Curry

Ingredients:

1 cup red lentils

1 large sweet potato, diced

1 can (15 oz) diced tomatoes

1 can (15 oz) coconut milk

1 onion, diced

2 cloves garlic, minced

1 tablespoon olive oil

2 teaspoons curry powder

Salt and pepper to taste

Preparation:

1. In a large pot, heat olive oil and sauté onions and garlic until softened.

2. Add sweet potato and curry powder, and cook for a few minutes.

3. Add lentils, diced tomatoes, and coconut milk.

4. Simmer until lentils and sweet potatoes are tender, which takes about 20-25 minutes.

5. Season with salt and pepper.

6. Serve hot.

Nutritional Value: Plant-based protein, fiber, vitamins, and antioxidants.

Cooking Time: 30 minutes.

8. Spaghetti Squash with Pesto and Cherry Tomatoes

Ingredients:

1 small spaghetti squash

1/2 cup homemade or store-bought pesto sauce

1 cup cherry tomatoes, halved

Fresh basil for garnish

Salt and pepper to taste

Preparation:

1. Preheat the oven to 375°F (190°C).

2. Cut the spaghetti squash in half lengthwise and remove the seeds.

3. Place the squash halves face down on a baking sheet and roast for 30-40 minutes until tender.

4. Scrape the squash flesh with a fork to create "spaghetti."

5. Toss the squash with pesto sauce and cherry tomatoes.

6. Garnish with fresh basil.

7. Serve hot or at room temperature.

Nutritional Value: Fiber, healthy fats, antioxidants, and vitamins.

Cooking Time: 40-45 minutes (including roasting).

9. Black Bean and Corn Salad with Avocado

Ingredients:

1 can (15 oz) canned black beans, drained and rinsed

1 cup corn kernels (fresh or frozen, thawed)

1 avocado, diced

1/2 cup red onion, diced

1/4 cup fresh cilantro, chopped

2 tablespoons lime juice

1 tablespoon olive oil

Salt and pepper to taste

Preparation:

1. In a large bowl, combine black beans, corn, diced avocado, red onion, and fresh cilantro.

2. In a small bowl, whisk together lime juice, olive oil, salt, and pepper.

3. Drizzle the dressing over the salad and toss to combine.

4. Serve chilled.

Nutritional Value: Protein, fiber, healthy fats, vitamins, and antioxidants.

Cooking Time: No cooking required.

10. Eggplant and Chickpea Tagine.

Ingredients:

1 large eggplant, cubed

1 can (15 oz) canned chickpeas, drained and rinsed

1 can (15 oz) diced tomatoes

1 onion, diced

2 cloves garlic, minced

1 tablespoon olive oil

1 teaspoon cumin

1 teaspoon paprika

1/2 teaspoon cinnamon, Salt and pepper to taste

Preparation:

1. In a large pot, heat olive oil and sauté onions and garlic until softened.

2. Add eggplant and spices, and cook for a few minutes.

3. Add chickpeas and diced tomatoes.

4. Simmer until the eggplant is tender, about 25-30 minutes.

5. Season with salt and pepper.

6. Serve hot.

Nutritional Value: Plant-based protein, fiber, vitamins, and antioxidants.

Cooking Time: 35-40 minutes.

These recipes are designed with anti-inflammatory ingredients and provide a variety of nutrients to support overall health and well-being. Please adjust the ingredients and quantities to suit your specific dietary needs and preferences. Cooking times may vary depending on your stove or oven settings.

Healthy snacks, desserts and smoothies for you.

1. Roasted Chickpeas: Drain and rinse a can of chickpeas, toss them with olive oil and your choice of spices such as turmeric, paprika, and garlic powder. Roast in the oven until crispy.

2. Vegetable Sticks with Hummus: Cut a variety of colorful vegetables like carrots, bell peppers, and cucumbers into sticks. Serve with a side of homemade hummus or other bean-based dips.

3. Almonds and Berries: A handful of almonds paired with a mix of fresh berries is a nutritious and satisfying snack rich in antioxidants and healthy fats.

4. Greek Yogurt Parfait: Layer Greek yogurt, mixed berries, and a sprinkle of granola or crushed nuts for a protein-packed and refreshing snack.

5. Baked Apple Chips: Slice apples thinly and bake them in the oven until crisp. Sprinkle with cinnamon for added flavor.

Smoothies:

1. Berry Blast: Blend mixed berries, spinach, unsweetened almond milk, and a scoop of vanilla protein powder for a refreshing and antioxidant-rich smoothie.

2. Tropical Paradise: Blend pineapple, mango, coconut water, and a handful of spinach for a tropical-inspired smoothie that's packed with vitamins and minerals.

3. Green Goddess: Blend spinach, cucumber, avocado, almond milk, a squeeze of lemon juice, and asmall piece of ginger for a green smoothie that's both hydrating and anti-inflammatory.

4. Banana and Walnut Smoothie: Blend ripe bananas, unsweetened almond milk, a tablespoon of almond butter, and a handful of walnuts for a creamy and filling smoothie.

5. Golden Turmeric Smoothie: Blend frozen mango, turmeric powder, ginger, coconut milk, and a pinch of black pepper for a vibrant and anti-inflammatory smoothie with a tropical twist.

These snack, dessert, and smoothie ideas are not only delicious but also packed with nutrients and anti-inflammatory ingredients that seniors can enjoy as part of their anti-inflammatory diet.

Conclusion

This anti-inflammatory cookbook offers a flavorful journey toward a healthier and more vibrant life. Each recipe within these pages has been carefully crafted to not only tantalize your taste buds but also to nourish your body with the essential nutrients it needs as you grow older. By embracing the principles of an anti-inflammatory diet, you are taking a significant step towards reducing inflammation, improving overall health, and safeguarding against chronic conditions.

The array of recipes, whether for breakfast, lunch, or dinner, will provide you with a diverse palette of flavors, textures, and wholesome ingredients. From the savory sweetness of roasted vegetables to the zesty kick of fresh herbs and spices, this cookbook is a treasure trove of culinary delights that prioritize your well-being.

But this cookbook is more than just a collection of recipes; it is an invitation to a lifestyle change. Embracing an anti-inflammatory diet means embracing a brighter and more energetic future. It means taking charge of your health, managing inflammation, and feeling your absolute best. So, let this cookbook be your guide, your culinary companion on this transformative journey.

As you embark on this path to well-being, remember that it's not just about the food on your plate but also about the choices you make daily. It's about self-care, self-love, and a commitment to a healthier you. Stay inspired, savor every bite, and relish the renewed vitality that an anti-inflammatory diet can bring. The power to live your best life begins with your next meal. So, let's embark on this journey together for a healthier and happier you.

Happy Cooking